DIABETIC CAKI

SIMPLE AND DE
FREE RECIPES FOR ANY
OCCASIONS

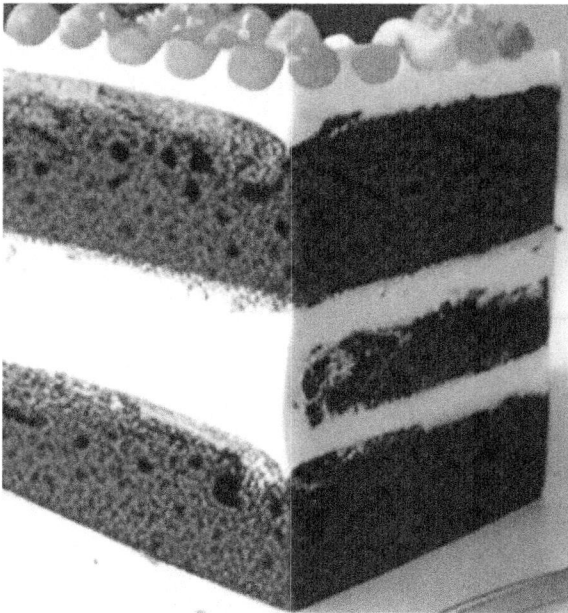

Dr. Malvin Harison

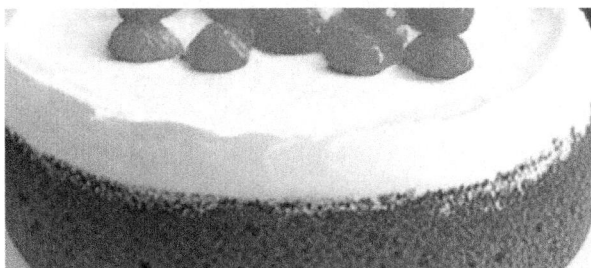

TABLE OF CONTENTS

Dr. Malvin Harison

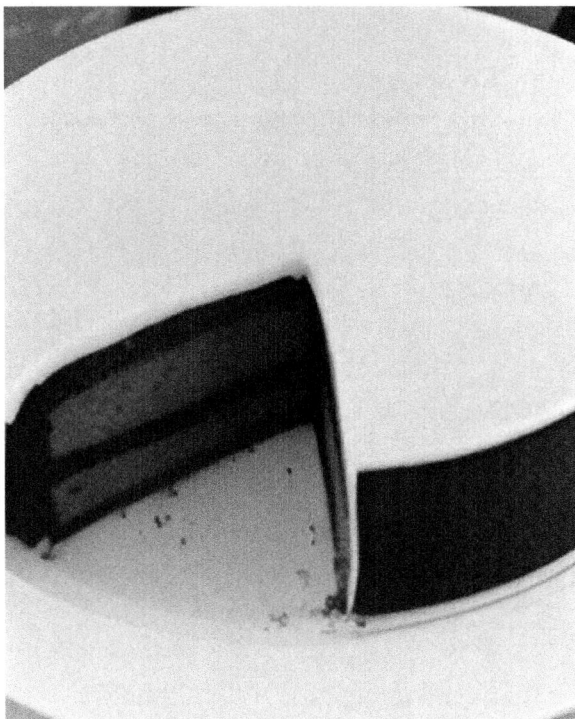

INTRODUCTION

Living with diabetes can be a challenging journey, especially when it comes to managing one's diet. For those with a sweet tooth, the idea of giving up desserts and treats can be particularly daunting. This book is here to help, never fear.

The Diabetic Cake Recipes Book is a comprehensive guide to baking delicious cakes that are suitable for people with diabetes. This book features a collection of easy-to-follow recipes that are low in sugar and carbohydrates, yet still packed with flavor and indulgence. Whether you are looking to satisfy your sweet cravings or impress your guests with a scrumptious dessert, this book has got you covered.

From classic chocolate cake, vallina cake to fruity upside-down cake, this book offers a variety of options to suit every taste and occasion. Each recipe is designed to help you maintain healthy blood sugar levels while still enjoying the pleasure of dessert.

So, whether you are a seasoned baker or a novice in the kitchen, The Diabetic Cake Recipes Book is a must-have resource for anyone looking to enjoy delicious cakes while keeping their diabetes under control. Let's get baking!

Cakes are a versatile and beloved dessert that come in many different shapes, sizes, and flavors. Here are some of the most common types of cakes:

Butter Cake: A classic cake made with butter, sugar, flour, and eggs, and often flavored with vanilla.

Sponge Cake: A light and airy cake made with eggs, sugar, and flour, and no butter or oil.

Chocolate Cake: A rich and decadent cake made with cocoa powder or melted chocolate.

Angel Food Cake: A fluffy and light cake made with egg whites, sugar, and flour, and no egg yolks or fat.

Red Velvet Cake: A moist and slightly tangy cake with a deep red color, often flavored with cocoa powder and buttermilk.

Carrot Cake: A dense and moist cake made with grated carrots and often flavored with cinnamon and nuts.

Cheesecake: A rich and creamy cake made with cream cheese and often served with a crust made from graham crackers or cookies.

Pound Cake: A dense and buttery cake traditionally made with a pound each of flour, butter, sugar, and eggs.

Fruit Cake: A cake made with dried or candied fruit and often flavored with spices and rum or brandy.

Mousse Cake: A light and airy cake made with whipped cream and/or egg whites, often layered with fruit or chocolate.

21 mouth watering diabetic cake recipes

1. Carrot Cake

Ingredients: 1 and 1/2 cups all-purpose flour, 2/3 cups of flaxseed meal, 2 teaspoons baking powder, 1 teaspoon pumpkin pie spice, 1/2 teaspoons baking soda, 1/4 teaspoon salt, 3 cups finely shredded carrot (about 6 medium carrots), 1 cup thawed, refrigerated or frozen egg product, or 4 eggs lightly beaten, 1/2 cups granulated sugar, 1/2 cups packed brown sugar, 1/2 cups canola oil, 1 coarsely shredded carrot

Instructions:

Step 1: Grease and lightly flour two 8x1-1/2-inch or 9x1-1/2-inch round cake pans and preheat the oven to 350 degrees F. Use parchment paper or waxed paper to line the bottoms of the pans. Oil and delicately flour the waxed paper or material paper and the sides of the container. Put away.

Step 2: Combine the flour, flax seed meal, baking powder, pumpkin pie spice, baking soda, and salt in a large bowl. put away. Eggs, oil, granulated sugar, brown sugar, and finely shredded carrots are all combined in a large bowl. Add egg blend at the same time to the flour combination. Mix until joined. Spread the batter evenly across the prepared pans.

Step 3: For 8-inch pans, bake for 25-30 minutes, or until a toothpick inserted near the centers of the cakes comes out clean. For 9-inch pans, bake for 20-25 minutes. Cool cakes in a dish on wire racks for 10 minutes. Place cakes inverted on wire racks. Cool totally.

2. Fluffy Cream Cheese Frosting

Ingredients:
2 ounces relaxed decreased fat cream cheddar
½ teaspoon vanilla
¼ cup powdered sugar
1 and ½ cups frozen light-whipped dessert toppings.
Instructions:
Step 1: Combine the flour, flax seed meal, baking powder, pumpkin pie spice, baking soda,

and salt in a large bowl. put away. Eggs, oil, granulated sugar, brown sugar, and finely shredded carrots are all combined in a large bowl. Add egg blend at the same time to the flour combination. Mix until joined. Spread the batter evenly across the prepared pans.

Step 2: For 8-inch pans, bake for 25-30 minutes, or until a toothpick inserted near the centers of the cakes comes out clean. For 9-inch pans, bake for 20-25 minutes. Cool cakes in a dish on wire racks for 10 minutes. Place cakes inverted on wire racks. Cool totally.

Step 3: In a medium bowl, beat decreased fat cream cheddar (Neufchâtel) with an electric blender on medium to high velocity until smooth. Beat in vanilla. Continuously add powdered sugar, beating until smooth. 1 1/2 cups of frozen light whipped dessert topping should be thawed. Lighten by incorporating about 1/2 cup of the topping into the cream cheese mixture. Add the remaining whipped topping by folding it in.

Step 4: One of the cooled cake layers should be placed on a platter for serving.

Layer a portion of the fluffy cream cheese frosting on top. Place the subsequent cake layer on the frosting; use the remaining frosting to spread. Whenever wanted, embellish with coarsely destroyed carrot.

Tip: Make certain to finely shred the carrots to keep them from sinking to the lower part of the dish during baking.

3. Breakfast Lemon-Blueberry Cereal Cakes

Ingredients:

3 cups antiquated moved oats

1 ¼ cups low-fat milk

½ cup unsweetened fruit purée

⅓ cup pressed light earthy-colored sugar

1 tablespoon ground lemon zing

¼ cup lemon juice

2 enormous eggs, delicately beaten

1 teaspoon baking powder

1 teaspoon vanilla concentrate

½ teaspoon salt

1 cup frozen blueberries, ideally wild

Instructions:

Step 1: The oven should be heated to 375°F. Cover a biscuit tin with a cooking splash.

Step 2: In a large bowl, combine the oats, milk, applesauce, brown sugar, eggs, lemon zest, lemon juice, baking powder, vanilla, and salt. Overlap in frozen blueberries. Split the combination between the pre-arranged biscuit cups, around 1/3 cup each.

Step 3: It should be baked for about 20-25 minutes or when a toothpick inserted inside it can come out clean.
Cool in the search for gold for 15 minutes, then turn out onto a wire rack. Serve warm or at room temperature.
Equipment Standard 12-cup muffin tin for making ahead Oatmeal cakes can be frozen for up to three months in an airtight container.

Microwave one oatmeal cake for 30 seconds at a time until heated through for reheating. Then again, refrigerate cereal cakes in a sealed shut compartment for as long as 2 days.
Oats are frequently cross-contaminated with wheat and barley, so people with celiac disease or gluten sensitivity should use "gluten-free" oats.

4. One-Bowl Chocolate Cake

Ingredients: 3/4 cup plus 2 tablespoons whole-wheat pastry flour (see the Note on the Ingredients), 1/2 cups granulated sugar, 1/3 cups unsweetened cocoa powder, 1 teaspoon baking powder, 1 teaspoon baking soda, 1/4 teaspoons salt, 1/2 cup nonfat buttermilk, 1/2 cups packed light brown sugar, 1 large, lightly beaten egg, 2 tablespoons canola oil, 1 teaspoon vanilla extract, 1/2 cups strong black coffee, Confectioners' sugar for dusting

Instructions:

Step 1: Spray a 9-inch round cake pan with cooking spray and heat the oven to 350°F. Line the dish with a circle of wax paper.

Step 2: Whisk flour, granulated sugar, cocoa, baking powder, baking pop, and salt in an enormous bowl. Add buttermilk, earthy-colored sugar, egg, oil, and vanilla. For two minutes, beat with an electric mixer on medium speed. Beat while adding hot coffee to the blend. It will be a very thin batter.) Empty the player into the pre-arranged dish.

Step 3: 30 to 35 minutes are needed to bake the cake until a skewer inserted in the middle comes out clean. Cool in the container on a wire rack for 10 minutes; Remove the pan from the heat source, remove the wax paper, and allow to cool completely. Before slicing, sprinkle confectioners' sugar over the top.

Note on the Ingredients: Because whole-wheat pastry flour has less protein than regular whole-wheat flour and is less likely to form gluten, it is a better option for making tender baked goods. It is available in natural-food stores and supermarkets' natural foods sections. In the freezer, store.

Tip: No buttermilk? You can make use of powdered buttermilk by following the directions on the package. or prepare "sour milk": Add one cup of milk to one tablespoon of vinegar or lemon juice.

5. vanilla cake

Ingredients: 3/4 cup fat-free milk, 1/4 cup butter, 1 vanilla bean, 3 room-temperature eggs, 1 and 1/4 cup sugar, 1 and 1/2 cup all-purpose flour, 1 and 1/2 teaspoon baking powder,

1/4 teaspoon salt, and 1 and 1/2 teaspoon vanilla extract.

Instructions:

Step 1: Butter and milk should be combined in a small saucepan. The vanilla bean should be cut in half along its length with a small, sharp knife. Scratch the seeds from the parts into the milk blend. In the saucepan, add the halved vanilla beans. Heat, stirring occasionally, over medium heat until butter melts and milk steams (do not boil). Eliminate heat.

Step 2: While the oven is preheated to 350 degrees Fahrenheit, lightly grease the bottoms of two round cake pans that measure 8 inches. Line the bottoms of the container with waxed paper or material paper; Lightly flour the pans and grease them. Beat the eggs in a large bowl on high for about 4 minutes, or until they are thick and light yellow in color.

Beat on medium speed for 4 to 5 minutes, or until light and fluffy, adding sugar gradually. Include salt, baking powder, and flour. Beat on low to medium just until joined.

Step 3: Eliminate the vanilla bean parts from the milk blend; discard. Beat in the vanilla extract and the milk mixture into the batter until well combined. Spread the batter evenly between the prepared pans.

Step 4: Bake for approximately 25 minutes, or until a toothpick inserted in the center comes out clean. Layers of the cake should cool for ten minutes in pans. Remove the pans' layers; cool on wire racks.

Tips
Tip: Choose Splenda(R) Sugar Blend if you want to use a sugar substitute. Follow bundle bearings to utilize item sum comparable to 1 1/4 cups of sugar.

6. Double Chocolate Cupcakes

Ingredients: 1/2 cups refrigerated or frozen egg product, thawed, or 2 eggs, 3 tablespoons butter 1 and 1/3 cup cake flour or 1 1/4 cup all-purpose flour 1/3 cups unsweetened cocoa powder, 1 and 1/2 teaspoons baking powder, 1/4 teaspoon salt, 3/4 cups fat-free milk, 3/4 cup sugar, 1 teaspoons vanilla.

Chocolate Frosting, 1/4 cup chilled 60 to 70 percent tub-style vegetable oil spread 2 tablespoons unsweetened cocoa powder, 1/2 teaspoons vanilla, 1 and ¼ cup sugar, 1 teaspoons fat free milk

Instructions:

Step 1: let the eggs and butter sit at room temperature.

Line eighteen 2-1/2-inch biscuit cups with paper prepare cups; place aside. In a medium bowl, mix together flour, cocoa powder, baking powder, and salt; place aside.

Step 2: The oven should be heated to 375 degrees F.

Beat the butter and vegetable oil spread in a large bowl for 30 seconds with an electric mixer on medium to high speed. Beat on medium speed until well combined, adding about 2 tablespoons of sugar at a time, scraping the sides of the bowl frequently. Use 2 more minutes to continue beating at medium speed.

Beat well as you add the eggs in stages. Beat in vanilla. Add the flour mixture and milk at the same time to the butter mixture, beating on low speed just until combined after each addition. The batter should fill muffin cups 2/3 full.

Step 3: Bake for 13 to 15 minutes, or until lightly touched tops spring back. 5 minutes, cool in cups on a wire rack. Take out of the cups; cool totally on a wire rack.

Hints: In the event that utilizing a sugar substitute, pick Splenda(R) Sugar Mix for Baking instead of granulated sugar. Follow the directions on the package to use the product in the amount of 3/4 cup granulated sugar.

7. Gingerbread Tea Cake:

Ingredients:
Two and a half cups of all-purpose flour, one and a half teaspoons of baking powder, one teaspoons of ground ginger, one teaspoons of ground cinnamon, half teaspoons of baking soda, quarter teaspoons of salt, quarter teaspoons of ground cloves, half cups of canola oil, quarter cups of granulated sugar, or a sugar substitute blend that is equivalent to ¼ cup of sugar, 1 and quarter cups of cold water, ⅔ cup full-flavor molasses
2 eggs, lightly beaten or half cup of refrigerated or frozen egg product, thawed, or

Confectioners' sugar for dusting
Fresh raspberries for garnish

Instructions:

Step 1: Spray a 13 x 9 x 2-inch baking pan lightly with nonstick cooking spray and preheat the oven to 350 degrees F. Place aside. In a medium bowl, mix together flour, baking powder, ginger, cinnamon, baking pop, salt, and cloves; place aside.

Step 2: Whisk the sugar and oil together in a large bowl until well combined. Add the virus water, molasses, and eggs; combine by whisking. Whisking just until smooth, immediately add the flour mixture that was saved to the water mixture. Pour into the prepared pan.

Step 3: Heat for 40 to 45 minutes or until a wooden toothpick embedded close to the middle tells the truth. Totally cool on a wire rack. Sprinkle the top with confectioners' sugar and, if desired, top with raspberries.

Tips

Tip: Choose Splenda(R) Sugar Blend for Baking when using sugar substitutes.

Follow the directions on the package to use the product in the amount of 1/4 cup sugar. Bake the cake for 30 to 35 minutes if using a sugar substitute, or until a wooden toothpick inserted near the center comes out clean.

8. Oatmeal Cakes with Cinnamon and Apple for Breakfast

Ingredients: 3 cups old-fashioned rolled oats, 1 1/2 cups low-fat milk, 3/4 cups of unsweetened applesauce, 1/3 cups packed light brown sugar, 2 large lightly beaten eggs, 1 tablespoon ground cinnamon, 1 teaspoon baking powder, 1 teaspoon vanilla extract, 1/2 teaspoons salt, 2/3 cup finely chopped dried apples, and 1/4 cup finely chopped walnuts

Instructions:

Step 1: Set the oven to 375°F. Cover a biscuit tin with a cooking splash.

Step 2: In a large bowl, whisk together the oats, milk, applesauce, brown sugar, eggs, cinnamon, baking powder, vanilla, and salt. Incorporate the walnuts and dried apples.

Split the combination between the pre-arranged biscuit cups, around 1/3 cup each.

Step 3: It should be baked for about 20-25 minutes or when a toothpick inserted into it comes out clean.
Cool in the prospect minutes, then turn out onto a wire rack. Serve at room temperature or warm.
Equipment
Standard 12-cup biscuit tin

To make ahead
Freeze oats cakes in an impenetrable holder for as long as 90 days. Microwave one oatmeal cake for 30 seconds at a time until heated through for reheating. Alternatively, oatmeal cakes can be kept in the refrigerator for up to two days in an airtight container.

9. Double Chocolate Cupcakes:

Ingredients: ½ cup refrigerated or frozen egg item, defrosted, or 2 eggs
3 tablespoons of butter
1 ⅓ cups cake flour or 1 1/4 cups regular flour
⅓ cup unsweetened cocoa powder

1 ½ teaspoons baking powder

¼ teaspoon salt

¼ cup 60% to 70% tub-style vegetable oil spread, chilled

¾ cup without fat milk

¾ cup sugar

1 teaspoon vanilla

Chocolate Icing

¼ cup 60% to 70% tub-style vegetable oil spread, chilled

2 tablespoons unsweetened cocoa powder

½ teaspoon vanilla

1 ¼ cups powdered sugar

1 tablespoon sans-fat milk

Instructions:

Step 1: For thirty minutes, let the eggs and butter sit at room temperature. Use paper bake cups to line eighteen 2-1/2-inch muffin cups; place aside. In a medium bowl, mix together flour, cocoa powder, baking powder, and salt; place aside.

Step 2: Preheat the oven to 375 degrees F. Beat the butter and vegetable oil spread in a large bowl for 30 seconds with an electric mixer on medium to high speed.

Beat on medium speed until well combined, adding about 2 tablespoons of sugar at a time, scraping the sides of the bowl frequently. Beat on medium speed for 2 minutes more. Beat well as you add the eggs in stages. Beat in vanilla. Add the flour mixture and milk at the same time to the butter mixture, beating on low speed just until combined after each addition. The batter should fill muffin cups 2/3 full.

Step 3: Bake for 13 to 15 minutes, or until lightly touched tops spring back. For five minutes, cool in cups on a wire rack. Take out of the cups; cool totally on a wire rack.

Step 4: Beat the vanilla, cocoa powder, and vegetable oil spread in a medium bowl for 30 seconds with an electric mixer on medium speed. Add powdered sugar in stages and beat until very smooth. Add sufficient sans-fat milk to arrive at the wanted spreading consistency (around 1 tablespoon all out). Frost cupcakes that have cooled with chocolate frosting.

Hints: In the event that utilizing a sugar substitute, pick Splenda(R) Sugar Mix for Baking instead of granulated sugar.

Follow the directions on the package to use the product in the amount of 3/4 cup granulated sugar.

10. Black Forest Cake Roll:

Ingredients: 4 eggs, 1/3 cups of flour, 1/4 cups of unsweetened cocoa powder, 1/4 teaspoons of baking soda, 1/4 teaspoons of salt, 3/4 cups of granulated sugar, and Unsweetened cocoa powder

Cherry Cream Filling: 1/2 cups of tub-style cream cheese, 1 cup of frozen whipped dessert topping, separated, 2/3 cups of chopped maraschino cherries, 1 tablespoon of sugar-free hot fudge ice cream topping, warmed, 10 maraschino cherries that have been d

Instructions:

Step 1: Permit eggs to remain at room temperature for 30 minutes. In the interim, oil a 15x10x1-inch baking skillet. Line the lower part of the dish with material paper; lightly flour the paper with grease. Put the skillet away. In a little bowl mix together flour, 1/4 cup cocoa powder, the baking pop, and salt; put away.

Step 2: Beat the eggs in a large bowl with an electric mixer on high speed for five minutes while preheating the oven to 375 degrees F. Gradually beat in the granulated sugar until smooth and lemon-colored. Mix in the flour mixture. Place batter in the prepared pan evenly.

Step 3: The top should spring back when lightly touched after baking for about 15 minutes. Turn the cake out onto a towel that has been sprinkled with unsweetened cocoa powder immediately after removing it from the pan. Remove the parchment paper slowly. Roll the cake and towel into a spiral starting on the short side. It should be placed on a wire rack to cool for 60 minutes.

Make ahead

In a little blending bowl beat 1/2 cup tub-style cream cheddar with an electric blender on medium speed until smooth. Thawed frozen whipped dessert topping in the amount of 1/2 cup; beat at a slow speed just until combined. Add another 1/2 cup of thawed frozen whipped dessert topping. 2/3 cup maraschino cherries must be drained; Cherry stems should be removed and dried. Mix the chopped cherries into the cream cheese mixture.

Roll the cake; Remove the towel. Spread Cherry Cream Filling to the edges of the cake. Fold up the cake and fill into a winding. Remove ends. Before serving, cover and chill in the refrigerator for two to twenty-four hours. Drizzle ice cream topping all over the cake just before serving, if desired, and top with cherries.

Tips and Advice: Splenda(R) Sugar Blend for Baking should be used in place of granulated sugar if you want to use a sugar substitute. Follow the directions on the package to use the product in the amount of 3/4 cup granulated sugar.

11. Chocolate-Fudge Pudding Cake:

Ingredients: 1/2 cup whole-wheat pastry flour, 1/2 cup all-purpose flour, 1/3 cup sugar, or 3 tablespoons Splenda Sugar Blend for Baking, 1/4 cup unsweetened cocoa powder, sifted, 2 and 1/2 teaspoons baking powder, 1/2 teaspoons salt, 1 large egg, 1/2 cup 1% milk, 2 tablespoons canola oil, 2 teaspoons vanilla extract, 3/4 cup semisweet chocolate chips, (optional) 1 1/3 cups hot brewed coffee, 2/3 cups of light brown sugar.

Instructions:

Step 1: Spray a baking dish that is 1 1/2 to 2 quarts in size with cooking spray and heat the oven to 350 degrees F. In a large bowl, combine the all-purpose flour, whole-wheat flour, sugar (or Splenda Sugar Blend), cocoa, baking powder, and salt.

Step 2: In a glass measuring cup, whisk the vanilla, milk, and egg together. Add to the mixture of flour; Using a rubber spatula, stir just until combined. Crease in chocolate chips, if utilizing. Scratch the player into the pre-arranged baking dish. Pour the batter into the measuring cup with the brown sugar (or Splenda Granular) and hot coffee mixture. Nuts, sprinkled on top. At this point, it may appear odd but don't worry. Cake forms on top with sauce underneath during baking.)

Step 3: The pudding cake should be baked for 30 to 35 minutes or until the top springs back when lightly touched. Leave to cool for a minimum of 10 minutes.

Serve hot or warm and sprinkle with confectioners' sugar.

12. Basic Yellow Cake

Ingredients:

½ cup refrigerated or frozen egg item, defrosted, or 2 eggs

3 tablespoons margarine

1 ⅔ cups cake flour or 1-1/2 cups regular baking flour

1 ½ teaspoons baking powder

¼ teaspoon salt

¼ cup 60% to 70% tub-style vegetable oil spread, chilled

¾ cup sugar or sugar substitute mix identical to 3/4 cup sugar

1 teaspoon vanilla

¾ cup sans-fat milk

Instructions:

Step 1: For thirty minutes, let the eggs and butter sit at room temperature. In the meantime, line two 9x1-1/2-inch or 8 x 1-1/2-inch round cake pans with parchment paper and lightly flour them; Put the pans away. Combine the flour, baking powder, and salt in a medium bowl; put away.

Step 2: Preheat the broiler to 375 degrees F. In an enormous bowl, beat vegetable oil spread and margarine with an electric blender on medium to fast for 30 seconds. Beat on medium speed until well combined, adding about 2 tablespoons of sugar at a time, scraping the sides of the bowl frequently. Continue beating at medium speed for two minutes. Continuously add eggs, beating great. Mix in the vanilla. Add the flour mixture and milk at the same time to the butter mixture, beating on low speed just until combined after each addition. Put the batter in the pans you've prepared.

Step 3: A toothpick inserted near the centers should come out clean after baking for 12 to 14 minutes. Cool cake layers in a skillet on wire racks for 10 minutes. Take the cake out of its pans. If parchment was used, remove it. Cool on wire racks.

13. White Cake:

Ingredients: 3 egg whites, 3 tablespoons of butter, 1 1/3 cups cake flour or 1 1/2 cups all-purpose flour, 1 and 1/2 teaspoons baking powder, 1/4 teaspoons salt, 1/4 cups 60-70% tub-style vegetable oil spread, chilled, 3/4 cups granulated sugar, 1 teaspoon vanilla, 3/4 cups fat-free milk,

Chocolate Frosting: 1/4 cups tub-style vegetable oil spread, chilled, 2 tablespoons unsweetened cocoa powder, 1/2 teaspoons vanilla extract, 1 and 1/4 cups powdered sugar, fat free milk is optional.

Basic White Frosting

¼ cup of tub-style vegetable oil spread, chilled

½ teaspoon of vanilla extract

1 ¼ cups of powdered sugar

fat-free milk (optional)

Instructions:

Step 1: Butter and egg whites should rest for 30 minutes at room temperature. In the interim, oil and daintily flour two 9-inch or 8-inch round cake dishes or line them with material paper; put them away. In a medium bowl, combine the flour, baking powder, and salt; put away.

Step 2: The oven should be heated to 375 degrees F. In a large bowl, beat the butter and vegetable oil spread for 30 seconds with an electric mixer on medium to high speed. Beat on medium speed until well combined,

adding about 2 tablespoons of sugar at a time, scraping the sides of the bowl frequently. Continue beating at medium speed for two minutes. Beat well as you gradually add the egg whites. Mix in the vanilla. On the other hand add the flour combination and milk to the margarine blend, beating on low speed after every option just until joined. Put the batter in the pans that have been prepared.

Step 3: A toothpick inserted near the centers should come out clean after baking for 12 to 14 minutes. The cake layers should cool for ten minutes on wire racks in the pans. Take the layers of the cake out of the pans. Cool on wire racks.

Chocolate Frosting: Beat the vanilla, cocoa powder, and vegetable oil spread in a medium bowl for 30 seconds with an electric mixer on medium speed. Beat in the powdered sugar in stages until very smooth. If necessary, add 1/2 teaspoon of milk at a time until the desired spreading consistency is reached. Frosting yields 3/4 cup.

How to Make Simple White Frosting: Beat the vanilla and vegetable oil spread in a medium bowl for 30 seconds with an electric mixer on medium speed. Beat in the powdered sugar in stages until very smooth. If necessary, add 1/2 teaspoon of milk at a time until the desired spreading consistency is reached. Frosting yields 3/4 cup.

Tip for Ingredients:
Splenda Sugar Blend for Baking is our recommendation if you want to use a sugar substitute. Follow the instructions on the package to use the equivalent of 3/4 cup sugar.
Equipment Two round cake pans of 8 or 9 inches
Prepare frostings in advance as directed.
Cover and refrigerate for as long as multi-week; Before spreading, allow to stand for thirty minutes at room temperature.

14. Key Lime Bricklayer Container Cheesecakes

Ingredients

⅔ cup crushed graham wafers (4 full saltines)

1 tablespoon spread, liquefied

2 ounces decreased fat cream cheddar, mellowed

2 tablespoons Key lime juice

¼ teaspoon vanilla concentrate

¼ cup powdered sugar

2 cups frozen light whipped besting, defrosted

16 slight cuts of Key lime

Instructions:

Step 1: In a small bowl, combine melted butter and crushed graham crackers. Divide the mixture into eight 4-oz portions. containers, squeezing softly with the rear of a spoon.

Step 2: Using an electric mixer on medium speed, beat cream cheese in a large bowl for 30 seconds. Blend in the vanilla and lime juice. Add sugar and beat until smooth. Overlay in around 1/2 cup whipped fixing to ease up the blend, then, at that point, crease in the excess garnish.

Step 3: Put the filling in a heavy plastic bag that can be sealed. Pipe the filling into the jars by making a hole one inch in the bottom corner of the bag. Place several lime slices on top of each.
Step 4: Put the lids on. Refrigerate the jars for up to 24 hours or tote them with an ice pack.
Carry the containers with an ice pack or refrigerate for as long as 24 hours.

Sugar alternatives: For this recipe, we do not recommend substituting sugar.
Equipment: Eight 4-oz.

15. jars with lids Upside-Down Pineapple Oatmeal Cake

Ingredients:
2 tablespoons light stick butter 1/4 cup packed brown sugar 1/4 cup chopped, dry-roasted macadamia nuts 4 slices of fresh pineapple, 1/4 inch thick (6 ounces), 1 and 1/4 cup all-purpose flour, 1/2 cup packed brown sugar, 1/3 cup quick-cooking rolled oats, 1 teaspoon baking powder, 3/4 teaspoon apple pie spice, ½ teaspoon baking soda, 1/2 cup buttermilk 1/4

cup canola oil, 1 cup refrigerated or frozen egg product, thawed, 1 teaspoons of vanilla.

Instructions:

Step 1: Place butter in a 9-inch round cake pan and preheat the oven to 350 degrees Fahrenheit. For about five minutes, or until the butter melts, place the pan in the oven.

Adjust the pan so that the butter is evenly distributed. Brown sugar in the amount of 1/4 cup should cover the pan's bottom. Sprinkle with nuts. In a pan, arrange the nuts on top of the pineapple.

Step 2: Combine the flour, rolled oats, brown sugar, baking powder, apple pie spice, and baking soda in a bowl. Make a well in the middle of the flour mixture. Add vanilla, canola oil, egg product, and buttermilk. Mix just until joined (the player might be somewhat uneven). Spread the batter out evenly over the pineapple slices.

Step 3: Heat for around 35 minutes or until a toothpick embedded the whole way through in the middle tells the truth. 5 minutes of cooling in the pan loosen the cake's sides; on a cake platter, invert. 30 minutes of cooling serve warm.

Tips and Advice: In this recipe, I do not recommend using a sugar substitute.

16. Quick Strawberry "Cheesecake"

Ingredients

1 and ½ tablespoons of graham cracker crumbs plus a pinch, divided ,1/2 cups nonfat plain Greek yogurt, 1 tablespoon strawberry jam, and 1/4 teaspoon lemon zest, divided

Instructions

In a bowl, layer yogurt, 1 and a half tablespoons of graham cracker crumbs, jam, and lemon zest. Add more crumbs on top.

17. Lemon Cheesecake Bites:

Ingredients:

1 cup finely crushed graham crackers; 1 cup sugar; 3 tablespoons melted butter; 1 cup fat-free milk; 1 4-serving package of fat-free, sugar-free, and low-calorie lemon instant pudding mix; 2 (8 ounces) packages of reduced-

fat cream cheese, softened; 1 (8 ounces) package of fat-free cream cheese, softened; 1/4 cup plain fat-free Greek yogurt; 1/4 teaspoon salt; 3 eggs, 2 tablespoons of finely shredded lemon peel

2 tablespoons of lemon extract

2 tablespoons of white baking pieces

½ teaspoon of shortening

2 tablespoons of pistachio nuts, chopped

Instructions:

Step 1: Preheat the broiler to 325 degrees F. Line a 9x9x2-inch baking skillet with foil, broadening foil over the edges of the dish. Place aside.

For outside, in a little bowl consolidate finely crushed graham saltines, 1/4 cup of the sugar, and the spread. Press evenly into the prepared pan's bottom. Cool for 10 minutes on a wire rack after baking.

Step 2: Whisk the pudding mix and milk together in a medium bowl until smooth. place aside. In a huge bowl beat Neufchatel cheddar and sans fat cream cheddar with an electric blender on medium to high velocity for 30 seconds. Combine the yogurt, pudding mixture, and salt with the remaining 3/4 cup of sugar.

Beat until consolidated. Beat well after each addition of eggs as they are added one at a time. Add the lemon juice and 1 tablespoon of the lemon peel and beat until combined.

Step 3: Spread the batter evenly over the cooled graham cracker crust. Bake for 65 to 75 minutes, or until the center still jiggles when gently shaken and a 1-inch area around the outside edges appears set. Place on a wire rack to cool in the pan.

Make sure the plastic wrap touches the cheesecake's surface before covering it with plastic wrap to prevent condensation. Chill for no less than 8 hours or as long as 24 hours.

Step 4: Combine the shortening and white baking pieces in a small microwave-safe bowl. Microwave on 100% power (high) for 10 to 60 seconds or until liquefied, mixing at regular intervals.

Spread the melted mixture evenly over the baked cheesecake; Sprinkle with pistachio crumbs. Lift the uncut cheesecake out of the pan by using the foil's edges. Divide into 25 pieces. Sprinkle with the remaining lemon peel, 1 tablespoon.

18. Matcha Castella Cake:

Ingredients:

6 large eggs, 3/4 cup, 2 tablespoons granulated sugar, 1/2 teaspoon mizuame, 1/4 cup hot water, 1 and 1/2 cup bread flour, and 2 teaspoons matcha powder.

Instructions:

Step 1: Preheat the stove to 325°F. Line two loaf pans (8 1/2 by 4 1/2 inches) with parchment paper and spray them with cooking spray. On the two sides leave a 2- inch overhang.

Step 2: Place eggs and sugar in the bowl of a stand blender fitted with a whisk connection; beat for about ten minutes at a medium-low speed until it has tripled in size and is stable.

Step 3: In a small bowl, combine mizuame and hot water; mix well with a whisk. After lowering the mixer's speed to low, gradually incorporate the mizuame mixture into the batter, beating for about 30 seconds.

Step 4: In a medium bowl, mix the matcha and flour together. Whisk completely to circulate air through and separate any clusters. In three clusters, add the flour combination to the blend in the blender bowl; beat at a low speed, waiting approximately one minute before adding more.

Step 5: Divide the batter among the prepared pans evenly. Lift each dish a couple of creeps over the work surface and drop it down to scatter any air pockets in the player. To eliminate any remaining bubbles, draw a zigzag pattern through the batter with a chopstick. 45 to 50 minutes or until a cake tester inserted in the middle comes out clean and the top is a deep brown color

Step 6: Use the parchment overhang to remove the cakes from the pans and place them on plastic wrap. Wrap firmly to seal in dampness; refrigerate for 8 to 12 hours. Eliminate and dispose of the saran wrap and material paper prior to serving. Serve chilled or at room temperature after slicing.

19. Blueberry Lemon Curd Ice Cream Cake

Nonstick cooking spray

Ingredients

1 16-ounce box of sugar-free yellow cake mix 1 cup water 3 eggs 1/4 cups canola oil 1 tablespoon lemon zest 1/2 (10 ounces) jar of lemon curd 4 cups slightly softened no-sugar-added vanilla ice cream, 1 cup assorted fresh berries

Instructions:

Step 1: Coat a 10-inch springform pan lightly with cooking spray and heat it to 325 degrees F. Use parchment paper to line.

Step 2: In an enormous bowl join the cake blend, water, eggs, oil, and lemon zing. For two minutes, beat with a mixer on medium speed. Put the batter in the pan you prepared. A toothpick inserted in the middle of the cake should come out clean after 35 to 38 minutes of baking. Cool in a skillet on a wire rack.

Step 3: Spread lemon curd over top of the cake; smooth the top by spooning ice cream over the lemon curd. Cover and freeze for eight hours or overnight.

Step 4: Eliminate from the cooler, let it represent 5 minutes before eliminating the sides of the skillet. Top with berries.

20. Mini No-Bake Pumpkin Cheesecakes:

Ingredients: 3/4 cup graham cracker crumbs (about 5 sheets), 2 tablespoons vegetable oil, 1 tablespoon honey, 1 tablespoon unsalted butter, melted, 1/2 cup nonfat cottage cheese, 4 ounces reduced-fat cream cheese, at room temperature, 1/2 cups nonfat plain Greek yogurt, 1/2 cups unseasoned pumpkin puree, 1/4 cups packed brown sugar, 1 teaspoon pumpkin pie spice, 1 teaspoons of vanilla derivatives.

Instructions

Step 1: Silicone liners can be used to line a 12-cup muffin pan, or you can use paper liners and spray them with cooking spray.

Step 2: In a medium bowl, combine the butter, honey, oil, and graham cracker crumbs. Add approximately one tablespoon of the mixture to each prepared cup. Pat down with clean fingers or the back of a spoon. Set aside for one hour.

Step 3: In the meantime, join curds, cream cheddar, yogurt, pumpkin, earthy-colored sugar, pumpkin pie flavor, and vanilla in a food processor; process until smooth, scratching down the sides on a case-by-case basis.

Step 4: Spread the filling out evenly between the cups, about 2 tablespoons per cup, and smooth it out with a spoon or offset spatula. Freeze for somewhere around 2 hours and as long as 2 days. The cheesecakes should be taken out of the muffin pan. Place the cheesecakes on a serving plate or tray after removing the liners. Before serving, allow it to stand for 30 minutes at room temperature.

To make ahead

Freeze for as long as 2 days. Before serving, allow it to stand for 30 minutes at room temperature.

21. Pumpkin Sheet Cake with Cream Cheese Frosting:

Ingredients:

One cup of whole-wheat pastry flour; one cup of all-purpose flour; one tablespoon of pumpkin pie spice; 2 teaspoons baking powder; 1 teaspoon baking soda; 1 teaspoon kosher salt; 1 cup unseasoned pumpkin puree; 3/4 cup water; 3/4 cups granulated sugar; 1/4 cups packed brown sugar; 1/4 cup vegetable oil; 1 and 1/2 teaspoons divided vanilla extract; 4 ounces reduced-fat cream cheese; 2 tablespoons unsalted butter, 2 cups of confectioners sugar, divided

Instructions:

Step 1: Preheat stove to 350°F. Allow parchment paper to hang over the edges of a 9-by-13-inch metal baking pan as a liner. Spray cooking spray all over.

Step 2: In a large bowl, combine the pumpkin pie spice, all-purpose flour, pastry flour, baking powder, baking soda, and salt. Add pumpkin, water, granulated sugar, earthy-colored sugar, oil, and 1/2 teaspoon vanilla;
whisk until combined. Spread the batter evenly into the pan that has been prepared. 25 to 30 minutes or until a toothpick inserted in the middle comes out clean. Before frosting, allow the cake to cool completely on a wire rack for one hour in the pan.

Step 3: In a medium bowl, combine the butter and cream cheese; beat on high speed with an electric mixer until smooth. Add 1/2 cup confectioners' sugar gradually; blend by beating at a medium speed. Add the remaining 1 teaspoon of vanilla and another 1/2 cup of confectioners' sugar; beat to blend. The remaining 1 cup of confectioners' sugar should be added; beat at a high speed until fluffy and smooth. Over the cooled cake, spread the frosting in an even layer.

22. Dark Backwoods Fro-Yo Cupcakes

Ingredients

1 ½ cups chocolate snaps, like Mi-Del (around 4 ounces)

2 tablespoons softened margarine

2 pints nonfat vanilla frozen yogurt, relaxed (4 cups)

1 cup slashed pitted cherries, new or frozen

2 tablespoons of scaled-down chocolate chips, in addition to something else for decoration.

Instructions:

Step 1 of Instructions: Liberally cover a 12-cup biscuit tin with a cooking shower.

Step 2: In a food processor, process the cookies until fine crumbs form. Mix in the melted butter in a medium bowl after transferring. Each muffin cup should have about one tablespoon of the mixture pressed into the bottom.

Step 3: Consolidate frozen yogurt, cherries, and 2 tablespoons chocolate chips in an enormous bowl and mix until very much joined. A generous quarter cup of the mixture should go into each muffin cup. If desired, sprinkle a few chips on top. Freeze until firm, something like 3 hours.

Tips and Tools: 12-cup biscuit tin.

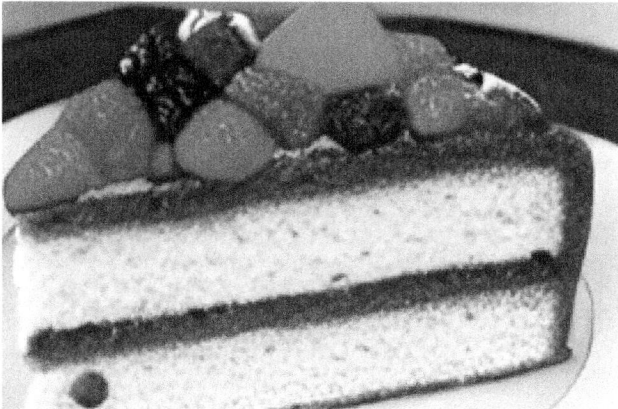

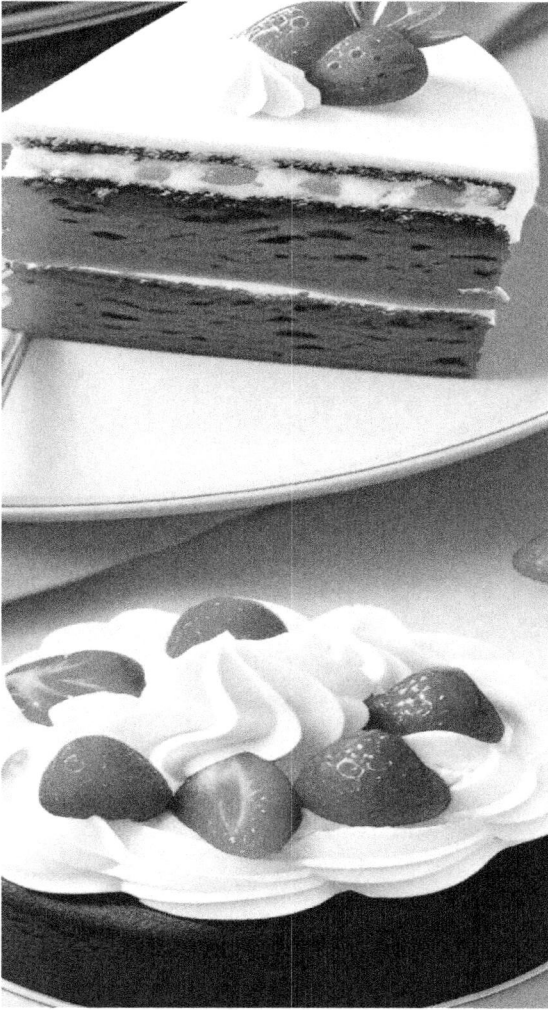

Printed in Great Britain
by Amazon

22962798R00030